I0827791

FOOD AS A PRESCRIPTION

A Handbook for Those Currently On or Prescribed a Gluten-Free, Soy-Free, Corn-Free and/or Dairy-Free Diet

Anthony & Staci Lo Cascio

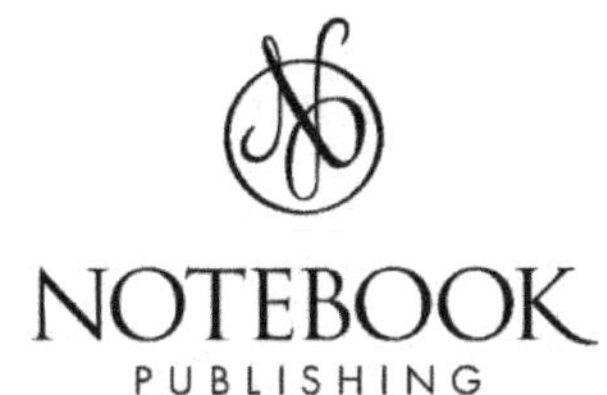
NOTEBOOK
PUBLISHING

First published in 2021 by Notebook Publishing of Notebook Group Limited, 20–22 Wenlock Road, London, N1 7GU.

www.notebookpublishing.com

ISBN: 9781913206451

A CIP catalogue record for this book is available from the British Library.

Typeset by Notebook Publishing.

We dedicate this book to you, the reader. May you discover something new that puts you or keeps you on a path to a better way of life. Food as a prescription may not be the answer to everything, but it certainly seems like the answer to many things. Use this book on your path to good health: to calm yourself; to find yourself; to heal yourself; and to discover what you may need for yourself.

If you ever have any questions or need guidance, please don't hesitate to reach out. Feel free to send us an email or a DM via our social media listed at the end of this book.

ABOUT THE AUTHORS

GREETINGS! WE ARE ANTHONY and Staci, two professional dancers whose lives and careers were put in jeopardy as a result of the food we were eating. By changing what we put in or on ourselves, we were led to experience food as a prescription.

This shift in mentality and lifestyle drastically improved the quality of our lives, and, by sharing our experiences and the knowledge we've gained over the course of many years, we will expose you to a wealth of information, in turn helping you to avoid making a lot of the same mistakes we did.

WHAT THEY'RE SAYING ABOUT FOOD AS A PRESCRIPTION

Anthony and Staci changed my life forever! While visiting me and my family in CA, they taught us the benefits of food as a prescription. We went food shopping together and they shared with us some of their healthy cooking. Wow! And so *much flavor. I am forever indebted to them!*

—Mike H. (Environmental Health and Safety Manager and Dance Dad)

Staci and Anthony bring me balance.

—Kristin I. (Small Business Owner)

Anthony truly is an incredible human being. The world can be a very easy place... to drown [in], and his bright light can pull others through darkness and save them from drowning. He helped me [to] see good things in people and find good things in myself; how to focus on the positive. This mindset has helped me come through to the other side more than once in life.

—Robby L. (Computer Engineer)

I started tap dancing as an adult, barely fresh out of college. I wanted to try something new and outside my comfort zone. In my efforts to find a beginning class at a good time, I eventually ended up in Anthony's class, and I continued to take [it] for over ten years until he moved out of the area. Anthony has had a positive impact on my life, as a teacher and as a friend. Even though I lacked rhythm and coordination when I started dancing, Anthony did not lower his expectations of me, and he continuously made me work; he was patient, and would take time to adapt his teaching tactics to fit the moment. He also helped me stay positive and cope with my frustration, which seemed constant at times! Tap dancing is hard—[and] it's really hard for someone who lacks dance experience. I eventually learned, but I would have quit over and over again if I [hadn't had] the opportunity to dance with someone who believed in his students and saw their potential to be the best they can be. I have been tap dancing for nearly two decades now, and I owe a lot of this to Anthony. This is just a tiny snippet of the positive impact he's had on my life.

—Ellen M. (Paralegal and Tap Dancer)

FOREWORD BY DR. ROBERT GUCCIARDO

IN MY JOURNEY AS a chiropractor and nutritionist, the one thing I have realized lacks in the patients I work with is the knowledge of food, as well as the many impacts it can have on our health.

There is a lot of data and misinformation out in the public, and so our job as humans is to search for and study the *useful* information that's out there so we can all contribute to the fight for our health and lives. We can either fight against things, or we can fight for things—and I choose to fight for something greater in life. I believe Staci and Anthony also share the same philosophy.

With knowledge comes understanding; with understanding comes wisdom; and with wisdom, we can share what we know with others and try to create a healthier world. I've known Anthony for a long time, and know that he has a heart for seeing others flourish. With the health journey he has been on with Staci these past few years, he has applied the knowledge he possesses in a way that will allow him to move forward—and now, he wants to help others gain control of their health.

Eating is purposeful, and we need to listen to our bodies. There are foods that we may be currently eating that are causing inflammation and stress in the body, and, if we continue to eat these foods, we will decrease our health potential.

In this book, you'll find solutions for implementing new, more healthful dietary habits. This book is about a fight for health, and such a fight is won by using food as your prescription. I hope and pray that this book is the prescription you need in order to change the course of your health journey.

Thank you to Anthony and Staci for your passion and desire—not just for your own health, but for the health of humanity as a whole.

CONTENTS

THE BIGGER PICTURE AND WHAT TO EXPECT

HAVE YOU BEEN SUSPICIOUS as to what your diet is doing to your health? Have you seen someone (i.e. a doctor; a chiropractor; a nutritionist; etc.) who has given you a "prescription" to change your diet? If someone has told you that you should eliminate gluten, soy, corn, dairy or other food group(s) from your diet, then this book is just what you need, and might very well become your best companion. When starting on a food- or allergens-elimination journey, advice from people who have been there is incredibly valuable. Their knowledge and experience will ultimately save you time, money, and, in some cases, your sanity! In other cases, it can even save your life.

Wrapping your mind around having to eliminate gluten, corn, soy, dairy, and/or other allergens may prove difficult, and doesn't just happen overnight. Implementing such a "prescription" can be both emotionally and mentally overwhelming, but we've got you covered! There are *tons* of support systems out there, and this book is one of them. As you read on, you'll find more than just some tips and tricks on how to navigate this lifestyle change. You'll find anecdotes, suggestions, things *we* wish we had known from the get-go, some of our favorite recipes, and so much more!

Personal Tip: Read the ingredients of *everything*. Make this your favorite new habit! If you can't pronounce an ingredient or don't know what it is or does, Google it—or simply don't buy the product. Implementing this one new habit will drastically improve the ease of your journey when faced with eliminating allergens or sensitivities.

Notably, any information contained within this publication is done so because Anthony and Staci have a combined 20 years of experience in this lifestyle. It is not meant as medical advice; rather, Anthony and Staci are simply sharing their personal experiences. You should always consult with your physician before entering into a new diet/lifestyle.

CHAPTER 1

GLUTEN-FREE, SOY-FREE, CORN-FREE, DAIRY-FREE DIET VERSUS LIFESTYLE

Celiac Disease can be challenging, especially for a nine-year-old child. It has been four-and-a-half years since my daughter was first diagnosed with Celiac Disease, [and] I panicked: I was not prepared or familiar with CD. Anthony and Staci were extremely knowledgeable about Celiac Disease, and provided many practical tips for my daughter to ease the road and adopt the gluten-free lifestyle. They gave me advice on the best GF alternatives and where I could find them. Their kindness and assistance has truly changed our lives.

—Donna V. (Parent)

MUCH LIKE DONNA, YOU'RE probably having the same thoughts we did when we were told to eliminate the foods we had eaten and relied upon for our whole lives: *What happens now?*

Don't worry! This book is here to help you navigate that journey. Hearing that you have to change your food and lifestyle habits can be scary—devastating, even! Change, for many, is an uncomfortable thing. This is especially true if it is regarding the comfort or cultural foods that are currently prevalent in your day-to-day diet.

First of all, let's quickly address the word "diet". When most people see the word "diet", they think it means changing your food habits for a predetermined period of time and/or with the purpose of "losing weight" or "lowering cholesterol". People also tend to think that once they achieve this goal, it means the "diet" is over, and they can go back to their regularly scheduled food habits. However, once they go back to their old eating habits, the same problems and challenges arise again, meaning they are faced with a perpetual cycle that will probably never result in a long-term solution. It is only when someone realizes or embraces the idea of a "diet" being something sustainable, rather than something that has a beginning, middle, and an end, that you will truly break the cycle. In other words, if you start to think of this "diet" as a *lifestyle* change, you'll be in a much better headspace to continue implementing new habits and reap the benefits of using your food as a prescription.

In moments of struggle, just know:

- You are not alone!
- We, and many others, have been where you are now.
- You don't have to make the same mistakes we did!
- It's a process. It'll be frustrating at points, and you may want to give up—but don't!
- If you embrace the parts of this journey that are hard from the beginning, they can become easier and more enjoyable over time. If you approach this from a negative place, you'll have a negative experience. Likewise, if you approach this from a positive place,

you're more likely to have a positive experience.

Here are some key things we've learned on our journeys which might also help you on your own journey:

- Don't buy something just because it says "Gluten-Free" on its packaging. Rather, remember to practice your favorite new habit and *always* read ingredients. This will help you ensure the item contains no other possible allergens.
- Don't try to instantly replace your favorite things as it could lead to immediate disappointment. Instead, find new things to love.
- The safest food you'll ever eat is that which you prepare yourself. You *can* dine out, but it will be a re-learning process.
- You'll likely need to find new resources for your foods and self-care items.
- Nutrition Response Testing is our favorite non-invasive test that can be useful in identifying other possible intolerances.
- Remember, you're not going on a diet; you're changing your life. There is no such thing as a "cheat day". When you "cheat", you only harm yourself and slow down your own healing process.

CHAPTER 2

WE'VE BEEN THERE—WHO WE ARE AND WHY WE WROTE THIS BOOK

Anthony's Story

Anthony and I went to high school together, and I remember him fondly: always a smile on his face; always caring about other people; always making people around him feel his energy and positivity.

—Bradley K.

IT WAS SEPTEMBER 1997, and I was a tap dancer with a principal role in the show *Tap Dogs* at the Union Square Theatre in NYC. We'd just finished our New York run, and next up was five weeks of shows in Los Angeles before embarking on our first tour of North America. I was doing TV appearances, traveling in limos, dining at fancy restaurants, partying all over town, meeting famous people, and going to movie premieres. Life was really good.

Then, suddenly, something happened that changed my life. This would send me on a journey that has taken me to this moment: 23 years later, writing about how changing my diet/lifestyle saved my life and my career.

You see, I had already been in L.A. for about four weeks, and, into the fifth week, I experienced something rather weird and slightly devastating. Be prepared: this is not pretty!

I had a bowel movement that caused me serious concern: I saw blood. And not just a drop: *lots* of it. I looked down and it was like a horror show just happened that had come from within me. It was terrifying! On top of that, it was painful and nothing was solid. It was like the "Earth moved under my [seat]", and I had no idea what to do.

All sorts of things went through my mind in that moment, including the fact that I was there with no family, and I was only a few weeks into a contract to dance eight shows a week for the next nine months. There were, of course, other panicked wonderings, too; things like why was I internally bleeding, would it just stop by itself, and what on earth had started it in the first place?

Honestly, I was embarrassed to tell anyone; this isn't exactly an easy topic to chit-chat about with other humans. So, what did I do? After a short period of self-denial, I got over myself and went to my company manager. With her help, I was able to set up a visit with a doctor in the next city, and started hoping for the best news possible.

Being on the road and trying to find the right doctor to help with this situation was very difficult, especially in the late 90s. I remember the first doctor I went to couldn't find a problem; instead, he suggested that since I was a male dancer, I was probably gay and coming to terms with being homosexual. Because I knew this wasn't true, it didn't help me find any answers or have confidence in finding a doctor that could help. This event actually sent me into further denial about what was actually happening to me.

As you could probably guess, such a "diagnosis" definitely didn't help with my feeling lost with the situation, and absolutely sent me backwards in my journey. We were traveling in and out of cities very quickly, and, since I wasn't getting any worse and I didn't want to lose my job, I just kept dancing while quietly monitoring my problem.

At the end of the contract, I went to a string of doctors in California, where I was living at the time. This went on for months, and yet I was never able to get any solid answers: doctors put cameras inside me while they took guesses and jumped to what felt like all kinds of uncertain conclusions. There was talk of surgery, but never a diagnosis—and I didn't want to let anyone cut into me or play any type of guessing games with my body without a specific and certain diagnosis.

I had not yet been made aware that it could be the food that was causing this problem with my health, so I was continuing to eat all the foods I had always eaten.

Diagnosed at one point with ADHD, the first food "culprit" I eliminated from my life was High Fructose Corn Syrup. That definitely helped my mood, focus, and personality, and was the first time I'd used food to improve the quality of my life. I could tell eliminating this particular ingredient had helped me significantly, and, while I didn't know it yet, this wouldn't be the end of my journey with the idea of identifying and removing foods or ingredients that were making me sick or otherwise harming my body.

As far as dealing specifically with the internal bleeding, I eventually had a conversation with my mom. She informed me that my grandmother often had to deal with Colitis, which, in my mind, finally gave me some type of answer to my problem. With this in mind, I continued to live with the issues. However, over time, I started noticing that my body was looking and feeling swollen. I realized I just wasn't feeling or acting like myself anymore.

It wasn't until years later, after moving back to New York, that I met the person who is now my wife (and co-writer of this book!) that the story really heated back up. Upon her recommendation, I took gluten and dairy out of my diet. I even remember her mentioning corn and soy, and, while I wasn't really ready at the time to address such a large part of my diet, I was totally on-board with eliminating gluten and dairy.

Shortly after eliminating gluten and dairy, I noticed my body changing. The swelling was going down, and my joints were also feeling much better. The best part? There were moments where the bleeding stopped completely. This was a short-lived victory, however, because the bleeding was still ultimately off and on. A much better scenario, but still not ideal.

Meanwhile, I had been seeing a local Upper Cervical Chiropractor with whom I had gone to school and dance class with as a kid. He also knew my story, and, as a nutritionist, he recommended a Nutrition Response Test (NRT); he felt that this, along with some natural supplements, would be sufficient in guiding me to a long-term, well-rounded solution that could finally bring my intestinal challenges to an end.

I traded teaching him tap dance lessons as payment for the test and subsequent care. From that test, we discovered that my wife, Staci, had in fact been correct in her original suggestion: I needed to be gluten-free, corn-free, and soy-free, but I could put the dairy back in. And there it was: after more than 20 years of suffering, someone was offering me a potential long-term solution through my diet/lifestyle alone.

Along with these changes to my diet, I started taking some supplements that would help my body to heal from all the years of damage I had suffered. Having this test and the supplement program led me to getting amazing results—namely, they helped me to stop internally bleeding. I've never received an official diagnosis, but I did finally get a solution void of prescription drugs. Food was suddenly my prescription for better health.

I am happy to report I am still on my journey, and the results I have discovered have been life-changing. For anyone suffering or questioning how to conquer health issues, I wish the same life-changing successes to you!

Staci's Story

Staci was quite a positive influence on my life at a very critical juncture. She encouraged me to live life to the fullest after my divorce, and even convinced me to audition for a local community theatre company. She knew I loved to sing and participate in the Arts, so encouragement was what I needed to take that leap after many years of putting that "me" aside. She also inspired me to change some of my eating habits for the better, and I was able to find myself again. I'm extremely grateful to Staci for the positive role she has served in both my and my daughters' lives.

—Lynn V. (Teacher and Thespian)

Soon after I was born, I broke out into hives as a result of being fed dairy formula. I'd just started my journey into the world, and here I was, already in a reactive state! Upon the advice of an array of doctors, my mom switched to soy formula and bathed me in oatmeal baths—and, sure enough, after making these changes, the hives went away. This incident led to a diagnosis of Mast Cell Disorder. Thankfully, after this initial episode, the condition went dormant, but it wasn't the last time in my life I would live in a situation where my body insisted on attacking itself.

After a trip to NYC one year, I arrived home with a sore throat. It was different than any other sore throat episodes I'd ever had and some testing revealed that a specific strain of bacteria was present. I was prescribed Cipro, and, a few months later, I started having strange symptoms that I'd never experienced before; specifically mouth sores that looked like canker sores, but felt much different.

These symptoms led to more testing, as well as the prescription of many other medications. Ultimately, only prednisone succeeded in eradicating my symptoms. When the doctors read my many test results, they were at a loss with how to move forward. It was on one of these occasions that I was advised to see a Rheumatologist.

My very first Rheumatologist was from Romania, and, after discussing my symptoms and initiating further testing, she landed on the diagnosis of Lupus and C-ANCA Vasculitis. In addition to prescribing some disease-specific, Western medications, she advised me to try the Blood Type Diet. This was the first time on my journey that I had ever been introduced to the concept of using food as a prescription.

This prompted me to do some research, and what I found led me to believe that taking the Cipro, along with other multiple antibiotics and medications throughout my life, had led to my many once-dormant autoimmune disorders becoming active again.

At this time in my life, I was attending massage school, teaching dance, and choreographing musicals at a local Park District. It was hard to perform my job and be on stage while dealing with the side-effects of prednisone. Issues such as excessive weight gain and extreme fatigue plagued me. My illness was starting to affect my livelihood and enjoyment of the things I loved.

The fact that I was still having symptoms after continuing the prednisone and following the Blood Type Diet made me realize it was now time to seek some further answers. I confided in one of the friends I'd met through the Park District Theatre, and she advised me to see a woman in the area who did EAV screenings—a nutritional and environmental sensitivity evaluation.

After waiting six months to get the screening, I finally got in. The first thing the nutritionist said to me was, "You don't have Lupus; you have Hashimoto's." As I stared in confusion, she went on to reveal more. "I see your C6 and C7 [lowest two cervical vertebrae] are protruding. Those with Hashimoto's exhibit this."

This was a great deal to take in upon meeting someone for the first time. Nevertheless, we proceeded with the test and the results showed what vitamins I was deficient in, that I likely had the MTHFR (Methylenetetrahydrofolate reductase) gene mutation, what foods I was reacting to, and what environmental allergens were affecting me.

Finally, thanks to Barbara Griffin, NMD, CNC of Vital Health in Orland Park, IL, I had a roadmap to better health.

This is where my healing really started: I started taking a daily dose of vitamins and eating/eliminating certain foods and changing the things I was putting on my skin in accordance with the test results. Some of the major things I had to eliminate included gluten, corn, soy, and dairy, as well as many minor foods and ingredients. I was also deficient in specific vitamins that are required for regular bodily processes. After a few months, I was able to taper off prednisone completely!

This was a *huge* step in my journey! To have been diagnosed with an autoimmune disorder and made to feel like I was going to be "sick" for the rest of my life had been overwhelming (as an understatement), but after getting these test results and having a guide to implementing these changes, it felt as if a weight had been lifted from my shoulders.

After moving to NY a few years ago, about nine years into using food as my prescription, I started showing symptoms of illness again. This time, I decided to see Dr. Robert Gucciardo DC, CN, to get my own Nutrition Response Test. After doing this, the NRT revealed a few changes that needed to be made to my diet. It was at this time that I also started taking supplements.

While the above helped for some time, my body is ever-changing, and I was (and still am) aware of the fact that my puzzle may have more pieces than the average person. In addition to Dr. Robert, I recently decided to seek out a Functional Medicine Doctor after I saw a friend on Facebook™

check-in to "Westbury Integrated Medical Wellness". This was extremely intriguing to me, and I made a phone call accordingly. Upon listening to my story, Dr. Dashiff immediately ordered specific testing: allergy/sensitivity "prick" testing, bloodwork, and stool, urine, and saliva sample testing. It was clear that the tests he'd ordered weren't the "usual" tests as per a doctor's orders, so, in turn, it was clear that I was definitely going to get some new answers.

When the test results came back, it was revealed that I had over twenty times the "normal" amount of lead in my body. As alarming as that was, that wasn't the highest priority, given I was about to be going out of town for around three months. Rather, the first priority was resetting my gut health once again. I had been allowing too many borderline ingredients into my body, and I was paying for it. (Reminder: There is no such thing as a "cheat" day when living this lifestyle!) Two of the major things I had to eliminate were sugar and yeast: they were causing a tremendous build-up of candida in my system, and I was put on an elimination protocol.

At this moment in time, the biggest takeaway I can offer is that food has been my greatest and most effective prescription for good health. Using food as a prescription, rather than relying on medications, has provided the best results for me to date, and I intend to continue down such a path.

A Note From Us to You

In our experience, Western medicine focuses more on prescribing drugs to mask symptoms, rather than implementing proper nutrition or using food as a prescription to treat the root cause. You may be reading this book because you've come to the same conclusion, or have been given a diagnosis that indicates you, or a loved one, need to change your diet. Above all else, keep advocating for yourself and do whatever it takes to find the right doctors and solutions for you.

CHAPTER 3

KEY ELEMENTS—TESTING, FOODS, AND SUPPLEMENTS

Nutrition Response Testing (NRT) is a tool to be used in helping us understand which organs and systems in the body are working well [and which are not]. In addition, this test indicates what nutritional deficiencies may or may not be present in the body, while allowing us to find the things that are causing abnormal cellular function.

—Dr. Rob

Testing

SOME OF THE TESTS people choose to get include (but are not limited to) blood tests, genetic marker testing, EAV Screenings, and our personal favorite: Nutrition Response Testing (NRT). Additionally, you may undergo stool, urine, and saliva sample testing, and/or the "scratch" allergy tests. Some of these tests are invasive and some are not.

In regards to Celiac Disease (CD), there is a specific test that *is* invasive, and it is a requirement that you eat gluten every single day for a period of around six weeks leading up to it. To us, it seems problematic that someone would be encouraged to eat foods that harm them, just to take a test that tells them not to eat those same exact foods. Keep in mind that even if you get a negative result from this CD test, it doesn't necessarily mean you don't have a sensitivity to gluten.

A combination of non-invasive and invasive testing may be your best bet since both can offer different results and information. Having had the best results to-date from the Nutrition Response Test (see Dr. Rob's description at the beginning of the chapter), it is the one test we recommend the most when you need to delve further into what is happening to your body. Ultimately, we suggest you listen to your body. If you feel better when eliminating allergens such as gluten from your diet, do so. Tangible solutions can often hold more weight than a diagnosis or test results.

Both foods and/or environmental toxins can cause abnormal cellular function in the body. One specific abnormal function in the body is an inflammatory response that can cause a long list of health challenges and/or discomfort. To help identify what may be causing such an inflammatory response, we recommend people implement the use of a food diary. The Nutrition Response Test (NRT) can also record your response to specific foods or environmental toxins to see if sensitivities exist.

Having this testing done represents the beginning of creating an atmosphere for the body to work optimally. An NRT will introduce you to a lifestyle that helps you and your body to thrive. The ultimate objective is to remove any stressors or interference that your body or bodily systems may currently be experiencing. Additionally, an NRT can typically result in a "program" of supplements that will aid your body in its healing process. We will address supplements a bit more later on.

We understand there may be an overwhelming amount of new information to process, but remember, knowledge leads to understanding, and understanding leads to wisdom. This is, after all, what we're all here for—to support one another so we can collectively (or individually) live a life where we all get to thrive.

Should you need a referral to see a doctor near you for Nutrition Response Testing, please reach out and we will be glad to assist you so you can locate someone to help. Alternatively, Dr. Rob can be contacted here:

Gucciardo Specific Chiropractic
www.drgucciardo.com
Drrob@drgucciardo.com
(718) 845-2323

The results of your NRT are going to be very important, as they may very well be life-changing. Having these results will do things like aiding you in creating your Food Card (discussed in Chapter 5), which will help you to clearly and quickly communicate your allergies to others.

—Anthony

Once you've undergone your testing, you'll receive a list of the specific things you'll need to eliminate from your everyday life. This list includes anything you ingest (smell or eat), or put on or around your body. Your skin is your largest organ, and it needs the same care and attention as your insides do.

Here are some additional items that can contain possible allergens:

- Candles (many contain soy);
- Paper straws (may be made from wheat);
- Shampoos/conditioners and deodorant;
- Sanitizers and soaps (body, dish, laundry);
- Household cleaning products, air fresheners, and essential oils;
- Other haircare products (hairspray, dyes);
- Makeup, other beauty products (lotions, body sprays), and perfumes;
- Shaving supplies;
- Toothpaste and gum;
- Any prescriptions, vaccinations, OTC medications, cough drops, or vitamins.

If you have a question about any item, bring it to your nutritionist so they can test your body's response to it as part of your NRT. Over the course of our care, some of the items we've brought to our regular nutrition appointments for periodic testing include various probiotics, vitamins, broths, and seasonings. This resolves the question of what you *can* have after testing and gathering a list of all the things you *can't* have.

To further this, once you receive your test results (whichever test you choose to take), you should not focus solely on the list of foods you cannot have, but sit down and make a list of foods you *can* have. This will help you to focus on the positive side, as well as to know what to buy when at the store.

It will help you focus your cooking on healthier choices for yourself, and you will feel empowered instead of frustrated.

Here's an example of the list Anthony made of the foods that he *can* eat:

- Boar's Head cold cuts
- Uncured bacon
- Breakfast sausage
- Grass-fed beef
- No-hormone, pasture-raised pork
- Tea
- Garlic
- Bananas
- Onions
- Oranges
- Olives
- Lettuces (except spinach)
- Cucumbers
- Celery
- Carrots
- Cherry peppers
- Wild caught shellfish and fish
- Gluten-free pancakes and waffles (homemade, of course!)
- Various broths
- Rice
- Potatoes
- Apples
- Zucchini
- Ginger

- Millet
- Any of the brands mentioned in this book at the time of publication
- Chocolate (soy- and wheat-free)
- Nuts
- A wide variety of dry seasonings (except cayenne)
- A variety of oils (i.e., olive oil; avocado oil; sesame oil)
- Shallots
- Pickles
- Peaches
- Plums
- Nectarines
- Certain ice creams (soy- and wheat-free)
- Arrowroot starch and flour
- Tapioca starch and flour
- Coconut.

And here is an example of the list Staci made:

- Cucumber
- Cherries
- Eggs
- Sweet Peppers
- Rice
- Potatoes (not Yukon Gold)
- Onions
- Garlic
- Dill
- Dry seasonings (not paprika)

- Buckwheat/millet/teff/cassava
- Almonds/Pecans/Walnuts/Cashews/Pine Nuts
- Coconut (raw; oil; vinegar; aminos; flour)
- Cane sugar
- Blueberries
- Strawberries
- Olive, canola, avocado, peanut, sesame Oils
- Chocolate (dairy- and soy-free)
- Green beans
- Wild-caught fish (not salmon)
- Wild-caught shellfish
- Grass-fed beef
- No-hormone, pasture-raised pork and poultry
- Avocado
- Uncured bacon, ham, and pancetta
- Coffee
- Carrots
- Zucchini
- Yellow and Butternut Squash
- Spinach/Kale/Arugula/Other lettuces
- Radish
- Celery.

Food and Environmental Allergens and Self-Care Items

Once I started practicing my favorite new habit (reading all ingredients), I was surprised to read just how many products have High Fructose Corn Syrup in them. This includes cough suppressants/syrups and drops.

—Anthony

We both have major allergies to gluten, corn, and soy. Staci is also highly intolerant to dairy. Once you identify your own food allergies, we recommend that you do extensive research on those particular foods. Be well aware, these are more than just "foods". They are protein chains that can be found in all varieties of items and foods. Here are some general things to keep in mind about these particular allergens. We have discovered these over our many years in this anti-inflammatory lifestyle.

Gluten can be found in wheat and other gluten-containing grains (e.g., barley; oats; rye). In the gluten-free community, it is common knowledge that gluten causes inflammation in the body and is a contributing factor to a long list of other ailments and health issues. There are many books detailing the benefits of being gluten-free and how gluten impacts the body. If you're still struggling with the effects of gluten, or are not entirely convinced on how gluten can harm your internal systems, we recommend seeking out some books that specifically focus on those subjects.

Dairy is another major well-known allergen. There are a number of dairy-free options out there; however, some of them can also contain soy, or other possible allergens. Elmhurst 1925 has an excellent variety and quality of alternative milks, and our favorite butter alternative is Earth Balance, since they offer a soy-free option.

Reminder: While eggs can be an allergen for some people, just because they reside in the dairy section of your local grocery store doesn't mean eggs fall into the dairy category.

Soy comes in many forms such as tofu, beans (edamame), milk, oil, sauce, and lecithin. While practicing your favorite new habit of reading all ingredients, you will likely discover soy in items such as candles, mayonnaise, frozen foods, and chocolate products. For chocolate lovers, there are some great soy-free options that also don't contain dairy; our two favorites are Enjoy Life Foods and Hü Kitchen.

Corn might seem obvious to identify, but it (and its derivatives) can appear in places you may not be aware of. Remember to avoid ingredients with the word "corn" in it (e.g., High Fructose Corn Syrup; cornstarch; cornmeal). Some other major foods that can be derived from corn are citric acid, polenta, yeast, and xanthan gum. For a more complete list, we recommend you read The Paleo Mom's blog post on "How to Avoid Corn". She is definitely a favorite of ours.

There are many hidden forms of each of these allergens all around you. Some of these being ingredients, some being products, and others being foods. Additionally, we will share where to find them in more detail further into the book. We will also share with you more brands that we have vetted as being safe for us. The list here is long, and we don't want to overwhelm you. Everyone's list is different based on their own allergies/sensitivities. To get you started, here's a list of the more common and notable "culprits" you may regularly encounter:

- Citric acid (corn/gluten)
- Natural flavors (gluten)
- Carmel and other colors (corn/gluten)
- Malt (gluten)
- "Gums" (Carob Bean/Guar/Xanthan)
- Beware of broths and soups: most start with a roux, which could contain flour
- Processed meats (soy/gluten/corn)
- Condiments (soy/gluten/corn)
- Artificial coffee creamers (gluten/dairy)
- Candles (soy)
- Drinks, including alcoholic, can contain straight-up or hidden gluten.

Your best bet is typically to do an Internet search specific to your personal allergies/sensitivities. That is what each of us did when we made the initial commitment to our new lifestyles.

Supplements

There was a period of a few weeks where I was having some difficulty, but didn't know why. A nutritional consultation revealed I had a copper toxicity. Not really understanding where this may have come from, Anthony reminded me I had recently introduced copper socks into my life, and had been wearing them frequently. A few situation-specific supplements were recommended in light of this, and, of course, I immediately stopped wearing the socks. That change in my supplement program helped my body to drain itself of the toxin, and I quickly felt much better.

—Staci

There is a mixed bag of opinions and research out there about supplements. Personally, it's results that ultimately compel me: when I take supplements and avoid my allergens, I get results. That means more to me than anything I read in a magazine, hear on the radio, find on a website, or see on the news.

—Anthony

As we mentioned earlier, the results from your Nutrition Response Test may include adding a supplement program. We both take supplements made by Standard Process. Our Chiropractor and Clinical Nutritionist tests each supplement and its dosage during each nutritional consultation. At this point in our journey, we get tested periodically (at least once every four weeks or so), as well as any time that we feel something new or strange might be happening in our bodies.

There are many brands of supplements, and they are not all created equal. Not all of them work for everybody. You may only need them for a short period of time, or you may not even need any supplements at all! Changing your lifestyle may be enough for you. Life ebbs and flows and your body changes over time. Therefore, your supplement program will change from time to time, too.

CHAPTER 4

BENEFITS—WHAT THIS LIFESTYLE CAN DO FOR YOU

I'll never forget the day I sat down to watch an online conference with my wife about food, nutrition, and autoimmune disease. One speaker, Dr. Tom O'Bryan, specifically made me understand gluten in a way I never had before: he explained how the lining of our intestines is like a cheesecloth, and to not think of gluten as food, but as a protein chain. We're talking about what we put inside of us on a molecular level: a protein that, when it gets into your cheesecloth, could rip and tear it, allowing other proteins that don't belong in your system, into your system. He made me understand that this can cause your body to fight itself, which, in turn, causes issues classified as "auto-immune". Once I visualized how gluten can cause the tearing of the "cheesecloth"—whether you show symptoms or not—, something clicked in my brain, and, from that moment on, I knew I never wanted to eat gluten again. Understanding how it was hurting my system made me better understand how removing the culprit, or "poison", could benefit my overall quality of life.

—Anthony

In my experience, understanding the benefits of this lifestyle helped me to understand why I had to eliminate the concept of a "cheat day" from my life: "cheating" puts my health at risk, and makes me experience inflammation and other uncomfortable symptoms. It also prolongs my overall stress and recovery, which is absolutely not acceptable.

—Staci

IN CASE WE HAVEN'T made this clear yet, changing our lifestyle habits has led us to solving many of our internal health issues. We do everything in our power to live what is known as an "anti-inflammatory lifestyle". For us, this lifestyle is not just a fad or trend; the benefits are real and tangible, and entering into it with the right frame of mind helped us to embrace any challenges we faced, in turn effectively setting us up for success.

The benefits of an anti-inflammatory lifestyle, along with exercise and good sleep, may include:

- Decreased risk of obesity, heart disease, diabetes, depression, cancer, and other health issues;
- Improved blood sugar, cholesterol, and triglyceride levels;
- Improvement in overall energy and mood;
- Reduced symptoms of arthritis/joint pain, inflammatory bowel syndrome (IBS), lupus, ulcerative colitis, and other autoimmune disorder symptoms.

In addition to those general benefits, some of the specific benefits we've personally experienced include:

- Weight loss;
- Decreased joint pain with increased energy;
- Elimination of abdominal pain and internal hemorrhaging;
- Clearing of itchy, dry skin;
- Decreased anxiety;
- Decreased hair loss;
- Discovery of new foods and ways to enjoy them;
- A new awakening and understanding of oneself;
- Overall better quality of life.

CHAPTER 5

THE MORE YOU KNOW

I have frequently checked ingredients multiple times over the course of taking my vitamins and supplements. This has allowed me to discover they have sometimes changed so significantly that I must find a different brand.

—Staci

REMEMBER YOUR FAVORITE NEW habit? Read everything! The simple act of reading ingredients makes you wiser and more aware. This is just *one* of the things that we've learned and something we suggest you do to help yourself.

Ultimately, we want you to avoid making the same mistakes we made. Using the knowledge contained within this book should help you make better overall choices, which will save you time and money as well as some of your sanity. This includes some tips and tricks as well as the names of some products (in parentheses below), which we have discovered are the best choices for us.

Inside the Home

- General Cleaning
    - Be aware of the products you use, which could seep into your largest organ: your skin. This includes any cleaning products that you will come into contact with. You may wish to wear gloves while doing your household cleaning. The ingredients in dish soaps and dishwashing liquids as well as other surface cleaners may impact your sensitivities. We recommend both hand and automated washer dish soap (*ecover ZERO*) for cleaning dishes and multi-purpose surface cleaner (Absolute Green) for wiping down countertops and other household surfaces.
- Self-/Personal Care
    - Just like with general cleaning, you should be aware of the ingredients involved in your self-care and personal care items. You may need to change your soap, lotion, and hand sanitizer (Dr. Bronner's), tampons (Tampax Pure), shampoo/conditioner (Desert Essence, Giovanni Hair & Body Care), toothpaste (Desert Essence), ointments, hair dyes (Manic Panic), edible grade essential oils, personal lubricants (water-based), laundry detergent (All Free & Clear, Charlie's Soap), washer balls to replace detergent (J&R Essential) and dryer balls to replace dryer sheets (NuVur All Natural Wool Dryer Balls), deodorant (Green Tidings [Staci], Arm & Hammer Essentials [Anthony]), etc.

- Medicines, supplements, and vitamins (Standard Process, NOW)
    - This includes cough drops (Fisherman's Friend), cough syrups (Maty's Healthy Products), as well as over-the-counter and prescription daily medications, supplements, and vitamins.
- Kitchen/Food
    - Food Products: Just because it says "Gluten-Free" doesn't mean it's great to consume or be exposed to. Instead, you should read *all* the ingredients and learn where allergens (e.g., gluten) can hide. Good pantry foods include: nuts (if not allergic); chips (Utz Snacks, Siete Family Foods); GF pastas (Tinkyada, Jovial Foods); GF Pretzels (Quinn Snacks); Paleo Puffs (Lesser Evil Snacks); chocolate (Enjoy Life Foods, Hü Kitchen); taco seasoning (Bearitos); taco shells (Siete Family Foods); 100% maple syrup; brown rice crackers; GF crackers (Absolutely Gluten Free, Simple Mills); GF matzo ball soup; GF matzo; rice (Lotus Foods, Lundberg Family Farms); dry organic seasonings and vanilla (Simply Organic, Frontier Co-Op, Nature's Promise); local honey; Fairtrade organic coffee beans (ground fresh as needed); GF breadcrumbs (Aleia's); GF breads (Canyon Bakehouse, Little Northern Bakehouse, UnBun Foods); turbinado, maple, and organic cane sugar (Wholesome, Coombs Family Farms, Relative Foods); GF flours (Bob's Red Mill, Anthony's Goods), organic free-range chicken broth (Imagine Foods); organic

coconut oil both flavored and unflavored (Carrington Farms); GF cacao powder (Anthony's Goods); vinegars: both coconut (Coconut Secret) and apple cider (Bragg); olive oils*: both regular and extra virgin (La Tourangelle, Bionaturæ); other oils including sesame (International Collection) and avocado (Lombardi [Smart Foods]); coconut aminos (Big Tree Farms, Coconut Secret).

*__Personal Tip__: All brands of olive oil are not created equal. Know what you're buying. There are a lot of blends and counterfeit oils, and this could be a possible contamination point, making you sick without your knowledge. Believe it or not, our favorite olive oil turned out to be the Amazon brand.

- Fridge/Freezer: Responsibly sourced proteins, including grass-fed beef, no-hormone chicken and pork, uncured bacon, and wild caught fish. While these high-quality meats and wild fish are not always easy to find in our local grocery store, we have found the best bet for us is to order from our online sources. In full disclosure, we looked at a few options and ultimately decided to become members of both Butcher Box and Crowd Cow with regularly scheduled subscriptions.

  Want your own subscription? Head to Butcher Box and use our referral code link to get a discount on your first order: http://fbuy.me/qO2kw, or head to Crowd Cow and use our link for a special offer: https://www.crowdcow.com/lu8zymt3xfqg.
- Condiments, including soy-free mayo (Hain Pure Foods Safflower, Primal Kitchen Avocado), Jewish

deli mustard (Ba-Tampte), ketchup (Woodstock Foods Organic), and soy-free buttery spread (Earth Balance).

- Other: Alternative milks (Elmhurst 1925 [sweetened and unsweetened; walnut, cashew, almond, hazelnut]); sodas (DRY Botanical Bubbly); pickles (Horman's—void of artificial coloring); GF beer (Corona Extra); pasture-raised, free-range eggs; GF wraps (Siete Family Foods); non-dairy cheeses (Good PlanET, VioLife, Myokos); deli meats (Boar's Head, Applegate); and fresh organic vegetables and fruits.
- Freezer: Premade pizza dough (Wholly Wholesome), frozen pizzas (Against the Grain Gormet), sausage links (Applegate, Jones Dairy Farm), frozen fruits and hash browns (Cascadian Farm Organic), and GF chicken nuggets (Applegate [there is cornstarch listed in the ingredients, but these have proven to be fine to be consumed by Anthony]).
- General things to consider for cooking:
  - ⇒ Most GF breads are much better after you apply a bit of heat to them. This includes the Siete wraps listed above. Toaster ovens or a griddle are the ideal ways to do this. If you have non-GF people in your household, place bread on foil in the toaster oven so there will be less chance for cross-contamination.
  - ⇒ If your entire family/household residents will be observing your new lifestyle along with you, one

of the best investments you can make is cast iron cookware: get a few sizes and varieties, along with splatter-proof lids and heat-resistant handle covers.

- You may also wish to replace as many of your cooking utensils as you can; and, additionally, you can sanitize your current eating utensils, plates, bowls, etc. in a dishwasher, as long as the final cycle can reach 150°F. Anything porous, however, needs to go! It may be hiding contaminants or cause ongoing cross-contamination. This includes (but may not be limited to) cutting boards or sponges.
- We recommend buying a new set of pots and pans if you have done extensive cooking before making this lifestyle switch. While not completely necessary for all, we believe this to be the safer option.

⇒ If some of your household residents or family members will not be participating in your new lifestyle, you should have your own set of cookware utensils; and, ensure they are clearly labeled and stored separately from their items.

⇒ A little-known fact about GF flour versus regular flour is that you cannot overmix GF flour due to the lack of gluten. This will help when baking! Additionally, due to the lack of gluten in GF flour, the elasticity will need addressing. There are substitutes out there to help you get that elasticity including psyllium husk, ground chia and flax seeds, as well as a few others. (We are still experimenting with elasticity in our baking. More about our experiences on this matter in our next book, *All We Do Is Delicious Vol. 1.*) We have also found it is extremely useful to include heat-activated baking powder (I'm Free Perfect Gluten-Free Baking Powder) in our recipes.

- Technology
    - Everyone has their favorite form of social media to use and different social media platforms can house a wealth of information that could assist you while you develop your personalized, allergen-free lifestyle. You can use the same methods and ideas we outline below for any Internet/social media platform. The social media landscape is ever-evolving, and the following information was accurate at the time this book was written.
        - ⇒ Facebook™ can be a hotbed of information on allergen-free living if you know where to look. Simply search Facebook™ Groups for a particular geographical area and some specific allergen-free key words (e.g., "Brooklyn Gluten-Free"; "Celiac Tampa"). These are great places to ask questions and meet new people who can relate to your challenges! In addition to local groups, there are national groups, international groups, and groups that will help you focus on staying healthy while traveling.

We've found these groups to be very useful. Some are public, and some are private; some may require you to answer a sequence of questions, and some may not. Once you have joined a few chosen groups, spend some time exploring each group's content. We currently belong to a variety of FB Groups. They include, but are not limited to: Gluten Free; Gluten Free on Long Island; Gluten Free Travel; Gluten Free Celiac Restaurant and Food Club, NYC; Easy Gluten-Free Recipes; Dining Out with Food Allergies on Long Island (NY); Gluten, Dairy, Soy Free, Paleo, Organic, Allergy Friendly and More; Gluten Free NYC & North NJ Dining Group.

⇒ In addition to groups, there are also Pages, and, just like for Groups, you can do a search for criteria specific to your needs and/or interests to find the pages you may wish to follow. You can follow the pages of doctors, bloggers, commercial businesses, authors, bakeries, services, goods, and even everyday people just sharing their stories. You can follow our FB page by searching both "Food as a Prescription" and "LOCA Foods Inc."; we think you'll find this to be most valuable.

⇒ Twitter is another great rock to look under when seeking information for living this lifestyle and for connecting with others who do the same. A few notable accounts to follow are Gluten Free Watchdog @GFWatchdog, Dr. Sarah Ballantyne @ThePaleoMom (as mentioned earlier in this book), and Gluten Free FollowMe @GlutenFreeFM. Be sure to follow us at @LOCAFoodsInc.

⇒ Don't forget about hashtags! They are super helpful. If you're unfamiliar with hashtags, you can consider them the "Dewey Decimal System" for the Internet—and, if you're unfamiliar with the Dewey Decimal System, please go visit your local public library. To discover what you seek, try searching hashtags like #GlutenFree, #SoyFree, #DairyFree, #CornFree, #NutFree, and #Vegan. You can put hashtags into any search bar!

⇒ Ultimately, if you want to build your network of informational sources, scour the Internet for bloggers, recipes, podcasts, hashtags, and goods and/or services on Google™, DuckDuckGo™, Tumblr™, Pinterest™, Instagram™, YouTube™, Reddit™, TikTok™, or whatever is the hot, trending thing at the moment. By curating your own network of influencers, mentors, and educators, as well as a support system of peers over various platforms, you'll often be able to get answers to many of the common questions you may encounter on an everyday basis. Of course, nothing is a substitute for a doctor you resonate with, but having this network will remind you that you're not alone and give you a place to go for more immediate support.

- We feel that the "Find Me Gluten Free" app is a *must* for anyone adopting this lifestyle. We'll go into more detail on how we use "Find Me Gluten Free" in the next chapter!

When on Facebook™, I search for things like "Hashimoto's" or "Functional Medicine". Then, I follow those pages and join the groups that speak to me.

—Staci

Outside the Home

Some of the things I keep in my #FoodBag are various kinds of nuts, food bars that I can eat (GoMacro), chips or GF pretzels, small packets of almond butter, crackers, fruit, salt, chocolate bars, hand sanitizer, supplements for the day, reusable straws, packages of plastic silverware and napkins, and anything specific I need for any particular trip, like sandwiches or other to-go foods that may need refrigeration.

—Staci

- General Considerations: Not everyone is going to take your allergies/sensitivities seriously; we come across many people who just can't fully understand the severity of food allergies—especially if it isn't something they've had to deal with themselves on a regular basis. On occasion, we run into people who don't even believe an allergen-free lifestyle is real and they consider it trendy rather than life-saving. Unfortunately, this pushback can even come from inside your own family or household. Therefore, you have to constantly be your own advocate: if something doesn't feel safe, don't be afraid to walk away or say no. Some people may wish to go as far as getting a Nima Sensor, a small mobile device that detects the levels of gluten or peanut contamination in any dish/food item.

- New Habits: We've already told you about your favorite new habit (reading everything), and now, we introduce two other important new habits that will help you to more easily manage your allergen free lifestyle.
  - ⇒ Food Bag: Every time you leave the house, you should have a food bag to take with you. This is your allergy-free "go" bag, and doesn't only have to contain food! Having this with you at all times is the best way to be prepared for anything: you'll never be caught out of the house and off-guard if you do this.
  - ⇒ Food Card: We took the idea of a business card, switched the vital information to our allergies, and made Food Cards via vistaprint.com. This permits us to easily inform someone of our allergies/sensitivities when needed, and is given to restaurant servers, the host of a party, or any instance where it is imperative for the person

preparing our meal to have instant access to our allergies/sensitivities. Here are our cards to use as an example when creating your own:

Hi, I'm Anthony. I have serious food allergies & sensitivities. It is with your care I stay healthy. While preparing my food please change your gloves & be aware of cross contamination. You are appreciated. Thank you :-)

My ALLERGIES are Gluten, Corn & Soy

My SENSITIVITIES are
Tomato, Cabbage, Brussels Sprouts, Camomile, Watermelon, Broccoli, Cayenne, All Spice, Cloves & some Citrus

Hi. I'm Staci. I need your help so I stay healthy.

Things I can NOT have...

Grains, Oats, Soy, Corn, Dairy, Paprika, Tomatoes, Mushrooms, Broccoli, Beans (green OK), Tropical Fruits, Vegetable, Corn, or Soybean oils

Please watch cross-contamination & pretty please, change your gloves. Thank you.

I appreciate you preparing my food safely. Thank you for helping to keep me healthy

Things I CAN have...

Eggs, Peppers, Rice, Potatoes, Onions, Garlic, Dill, dried seasonings, Thyme, Cinnamon, Buckwheat, Millet, Apples, Blueberries, Strawberries, Olive, Canola, & Peanut Oil

Please ask about anything else not listed here.

Head over to this link to create your own Food Card: https://locafoodsinc.com/affiliates.

You have to start reconsidering every aspect of your life. Going out to dinner, visiting a friend, and going to a party will all be new and having a #FoodBag or #FoodCard will help in the ease of the process. Other things people can forget to reconsider is planning for a vacation or a road trip.

—Anthony

Here are some tips on how to ensure you have a good experience on longer trips such as vacations or road trips.

- **Where we stay**
  - Airbnb: By having access to spaces with a kitchen, we have found it easier to control our food situation when we're away from home with Airbnb. Having a kitchen allows us to cook our own food with our own equipment (if we choose to bring it) so we can stay safe.
  - Friends' Houses: Along our travels, we love staying with friends. Depending on the friends that you have, this would likely be the best option: similar to an Airbnb, you'll likely have access to a kitchen, where you can stay safe with your own food and cooking equipment while hanging with friends. As a thank-you, we love to cook for them, too!
  - Hotels: We only choose this option as a last resort. There are a few hotel chains that offer suites, which include kitchens. We try to stay in a room with a kitchen first, but this is not always an option. It has also become fairly regular practice for hotels to have a refrigerator in the room. You should call ahead to any hotel you reserve to confirm if there will be a refrigerator or not so you can plan accordingly. Sometimes, all it takes is a simple request.
  - Inclusive Resorts/Cruises: In this instance, we follow the tips and questions laid out in Chapter 6 under "Picking a Restaurant" to ensure we can dine safely. Speaking specifically to a chef prior to booking your trip will help you feel good about the

dining options the resort offers and if they can accommodate you. The last thing you want to do is get to an inclusive resort or onto a cruise ship and find out they have little-to-nothing safe for you to eat.

In cases where we don't have kitchen access, we tend to rely heavily on the Find Me Gluten Free app and/or a "Gluten-Free Farm to Table" Internet search.

—Anthony

Depending on how long the trip is, we either shop before we leave and fill the cooler or stop along the way. Often, it is a combination of both.

—Staci

- **What we bring**
  - Electric Refrigerator: Purchase an electric cooler/refrigerator for trips that will span longer than a day. Ours has an A/C adapter, so it plugs into the "cigarette lighter" in the car, as well as a standard wall socket. We personally have a Coleman Thermoelectric 40 Quart Cooler.
  - Cooking Devices: Bring your own selection of pots and pans and cooking and eating utensils if you're not familiar with what will be available—and, even if you're aware of the situation beforehand, it's always

best to bring your own equipment to avoid possible cross-contamination. We bring everything from spatulas to our crockpot depending on the trip.

- **General**
    - Speak to anyone you encounter along your travels. You never know when you will find locals or someone who has some great knowledge of that area and can offer pointed advice.
    - As long as you don't feel like your health will be compromised, stay open to new experiences. Isn't that what life is about?
    - This is a great time to use your social media skills searching terms like "[town/city name] gluten free farm to table" or taking advantage of the Find Me Gluten Free app.

CHAPTER 6

SAFELY EATING OUT—IN MORE DETAIL

A great thing to do would be to call ahead and speak to the party or restaurant host personally about your situation. Shortly after your conversation, texting or emailing the host a copy of your Food Card is an easy method of conveying your sensitivities.

—Anthony

IT CAN BE SCARY to eat outside of your own kitchen with or without allergies and sensitivities. Nevertheless, it can be done. Here are a few things we do to ensure we have the best experiences outside of our home kitchen; they will help to guide you as you venture out and about.

Going to parties at friends' houses, family gatherings, or restaurants, as well as "outings" (e.g., theme parks; jazz/comedy clubs; the theatre/movies), are all situations where you will have to plan ahead to ensure your health is truly in your own hands, ensuring the best possible experience for yourself from a food perspective.

When going to friends' houses or family gatherings, our advice depends on whether it's going to be a "friendly" or "hostile" environment, as far as the food offered goes. Does the host take your allergies/sensitivities seriously into consideration? And, do the other attendees take your allergies/sensitivities seriously?

If you can answer these questions positively, you should have a pretty awesome experience. Work with the host to ensure you have safe things available to consume, either without fear of cross-contamination, or with rules in place that create awareness for all guests present.

If you cannot answer these questions positively or with certainty, you'll need to plan ahead for yourself. Depending on the event and location, this can be as simple as bringing your food bag along. If you would like to bring something to warm or cook in the oven or on the stove, you should check with the host prior to your arrival—and, if this is okay, you may wish to bring all the things you'll need from your own uncontaminated kitchen (e.g., seasonings; pots and pans; serving dishes; and even utensils) in order to make the food you wish.

It's important to determine ahead of time whether you'll be consuming your food exclusively, or whether you'll be able to offer it to other guests, too. If you're sharing with other guests, make sure you politely make them aware of cross-contamination, and, if left unattended, definitely include a serving utensil that is exclusively used with the dish you prepared.

Having food allergies and/or sensitivities shouldn't exclude you from the dining out experience. Many people with food allergies or sensitivities enjoy going out to dinner and exploring different places and atmospheres to eat. That said, your health shouldn't stop you from partaking in this pleasure—plus, not everyone wants to cook every meal! Hence, finding quality restaurants that understand and care about keeping their customers healthy, whether they have allergies or not, can be challenging but not impossible. It can be difficult—but, thankfully it's getting increasingly easier.

We travel a great deal, so we have pretty extensive experience finding restaurants, eateries, cafés, coffee shops, health food/grocery stores, and bakeries in a variety of places and situations! Due to this, we have developed a method of consistently finding safe places to eat, whether this be on our own stomping grounds or traversing the country. We have acquired several favorite places we can now frequent in the process—something that took some time and didn't happen by accident, but was so worth it. After many phone calls, lots of questions, patient people, and chefs who were, first and foremost, interested in keeping us healthy, we developed relationships with the business owners and employees of what became our favorite restaurants both locally and nationally. The approach, mindset, and methods, more often than not, provide us with great experiences and keep us safe.

We want you to have great experiences, too, so we'll share our method of finding safe places to eat. This information will help you learn about our process so you can successfully go out and have wonderful dining experiences while building your own network of safe spaces to frequent.

Picking a Restaurant/Bakery/Eatery

Before calling, I like to remind myself to be kind, be considerate, and to be sure to get a name. I also try to call during "off hours" so I can be very thorough—which can take some time. These are my responsibilities. This is my health challenge and not someone else's.

—Anthony

From now on, you may have to be the one that always picks the restaurant in order to ensure your safety. However, picking the restaurant will prepare you to eat out with friends and relatives virtually stress-free. We recommend you have a positive attitude when contacting any establishment: your energy will certainly have an effect on your experience and, ultimately, your food. Some places may be dismissive and that is fine. Not everyone has to "cater" to our allergies. Not every place is for everyone. Here is what we've found to work when picking a restaurant.

When starting a search for food, we like to begin with the app we mentioned earlier, Find Me Gluten Free. We use the search function by location, then set our preferred filters. One key filter is searching by what time you'd like to visit the establishment; another filter is if they have a gluten-free menu available. Some of the features are free, and some of them are paid (Premium), the Premium version coming with a yearly fee. We find the fee to be well worth it, considering the extra functionality the app can provide.

After narrowing down the list of potential restaurants, etc. we give them each a call, addressing the following questions and talking points. These particular questions are specific to our allergies/sensitivities. You should develop your own list of questions specific to you:

- Do you have an allergens menu?
- What type of grease/oil/spray do you cook with? Is the oil a blend, or is it 100% olive (or other) oil?
- Is there a dedicated fryer? If so, what type of oil does it use? What else goes in that fryer that may contain allergens? (E.g., If gluten-free mozzarella sticks are also prepared in the fryer, they can contain soy or dairy, creating a cross-contamination situation.)
- Are there specific GF items on the menu? Do those items possibly also contain corn, soy, dairy, or any other allergens?
- Is the chef willing to make something off the menu to accommodate [if there is not a GF option]? Is the chef available to speak with me before arriving at your establishment?
- What is the name of the person you're speaking to? Will they will be there when you arrive for your meal? If not, who should you ask for once you arrive at the establishment? Is there a specific server who is specially trained in handling food allergy accommodations? You can also ask for a long-time employee who may be more familiar with the menu. Would you like me to send you a copy of my Food Card? (You can get an email address or even phone number to text.)

Be sure to adapt your set of questions depending on the type of business you are calling. When calling something such as a bakery, ask, "What type of flours or sweeteners do you use?"

Whether the app returns anything suitable or not, we often also search the web for "Gluten Free Farm to Table near me". After narrowing down the list of potential restaurants, etc., we give them each a call and ask each of the questions listed previously.

Further, since you now always carry your Food Card, once you arrive it'll be easy to express your situation to your server simply by handing them a copy of the card before ordering your meal.

I find the wait-staff and kitchen to be very appreciative: they can just refer to my Food Card instead of making multiple trips to the table in order to confirm the things we spoke about.

—Staci

When searching for a restaurant, remember to read the reviews. It's just as important to read the 1-star reviews as it is to read the 5-star reviews (and all the stars in-between). If someone took the time to write a review, they obviously had something to say. You can learn a lot from other people's experiences. However, still use critical thinking and take what you're reading with a grain of salt. The overall star rating is obviously important, but be sure to compare that to how many reviews have been written in total and put the real emphasis on what the writer experienced.

—Anthony

Nothing in life is guaranteed, but following the outlined steps drastically increases your odds of having safe, positive experiences while simultaneously avoiding your allergens and staying healthy. The most important thing is not to settle when seeking a place to dine. Rather, you should keep calling around until you find some place you're comfortable with. If you get somewhere and start to feel uncomfortable, don't be afraid to leave. No one should ever fault you for not wanting to take a risk. This is about your health! In addition, because you bring it everywhere, your food bag is most definitely nearby or in the car.

CHAPTER 7

FOOD DIARY EXAMPLES

There've been many difficult moments along the journey of eliminating corn, gluten, and soy for me. Something that was hard early on was realizing I might need to throw out some food. By the time I got my NRT, I already understood the kind of damage certain foods were doing to me and might be doing to other people. At this point, I had a kitchen that was mixed with food I both could and couldn't eat. I started to realize the food I couldn't eat was now taking up too much space. At first, I was going to give the food I couldn't eat to my parents, but, knowing what I now knew about food, I felt like I would basically be giving them poison. Almost every item I needed to get rid of was already opened, so I couldn't even bring the food to a shelter. At this moment, I realized my only option was to throw the food away. It was slightly depressing and a very difficult thing to do as I was taught to never, ever throw food away. As I sat with this concept for a few hours, I realized just how sick this food was making me. It became more evident that, if I wanted to stop internally bleeding for good, purging anything that was making me sick was a necessary part of my healing process. I needed to fill my space with only foods that I could eat, and if there was something in my space that I couldn't eat, it needed to go. The good news? My positive approach quickly turned what could *have been a low point in my healing journey into a high point. Throwing that food away ultimately liberated me. I felt even freer later that week when I threw the trash out and realized there was nothing in my kitchen that could hurt me anymore. That was a beautiful moment.*

—Anthony

AS YOU GET DOWN to the bottom of your issues with any allergies and/or sensitivities, keeping a food diary is an amazing tool that can be very insightful. Looking back over a week's worth of meals can teach you a lot about your habits, as well as how you can possibly improve them. It will also help inform you as to what could be harming your health versus what is promoting healing. Be sure to keep track of any unusual reactions which can help you identify any possible contaminants.

Following is an example of a week of meals for both of us, along with snacks and dessert:

SAMPLE 1

FOOD DIARY

We recommend you use this #FoodDiary as a helpful tool on your journey. Visit our website at www.locafoodsinc.com to get a PDF emailed to you which you can print at home. While keeping track of your food throughout the day, be sure to also notate any liquids you consume and any environmental changes including new products you try.

Day 1 - Date: *Monday*

BREAKFAST *Time:*	**LUNCH** *Time:*	**DINNER** *Time:*
Scambled eggs with pancetta & onions	*Grass-fed burger w/non-dairy Mozzarella on Millet & gluten-free bun with lettuce. A handful of chips and some pickle chips.*	*Chicken cutlet w/dairy-free mashed potatoes*

SNACKS: *10 raw cashews, dairy-free and soy-free chocolate bar*
BOWEL MOVEMENTS: **Include shape/texture as well as terms like constipation, normal, diarrhea*
OVERALL MOOD: **Include words like happy, stressed, content, sad, focused, balanced, etc*

Day 2 - Date: *Tuesday*

BREAKFAST *Time:*	**LUNCH** *Time:*	**DINNER** *Time:*
LOCA Foods Pancakes & 3 sausage links	*Chicken nuggets, a handful of chips and a pickle*	*4 Tacos (Siete shells & non-dairy chedder)*

SNACKS: *15 raw almonds, handful of gluten-free pretzels*
BOWEL MOVEMENTS:
OVERALL MOOD:

Day 3 - Date: *Wednesday*

BREAKFAST *Time:*	**LUNCH** *Time:*	**DINNER** *Time:*
Scambled eggs with pancetta & onions	*Salmon fillet w/garlic green beans*	*Grass-fed filet w/potatoes & onions w/LOCA Foods "no-corn" bread muffin*

SNACKS: *Handful of potato chips, LOCA Foods zucchini bread*
BOWEL MOVEMENTS:
OVERALL MOOD:

Food Diary provided by LOCA Foods, LLC for Food as a Prescription - info@locafoodsinc.com

Day 4 - Date: *Thursday*

BREAKFAST *Time:*	**LUNCH** *Time:*	**DINNER** *Time:*
French toast w/maple sausages	*Uncured ham, herb turkey sandwich with avocado mayo*	*Marinated grass-fed skirt steak w/non-dairy mashed potatoes & steamed carrots*

SNACKS: *10 raw almonds, LOCA Foods carrot cake*
BOWEL MOVEMENTS:
OVERALL MOOD:

Day 5 - Date:

BREAKFAST *Time:*	**LUNCH** *Time:*	**DINNER** *Time:*
2 scrambled eggs with uncured pancetta & non-dairy mozzerella	*Gluten-free matzoball soup w/tinkyado shells*	*LOCA Foods lemon butter shrimp w/poached carrots*

SNACKS: *organic peach, LOCA Foods chocolate cake slice*
BOWEL MOVEMENTS:
OVERALL MOOD:

Day 6 - Date:

BREAKFAST *Time:*	**LUNCH** *Time:*	**DINNER** *Time:*
Grass-fed steak & eggs	*Uncured ham, herb turkey sandwich with avocado mayo and a handful of chips*	*Shared crab legs & LOCA Foods chicken wings w/lobster tail & rice*

SNACKS: *pasta salad, LOCA Foods chocolate chip cookies*
BOWEL MOVEMENTS:
OVERALL MOOD:

Day 7 - Date:

BREAKFAST *Time:*	**LUNCH** *Time:*	**DINNER** *Time:*
Frittata w/sausage, non-dairy cheese, peppers & onions	*Salad w/radish, cucumber, left over crab meat, LOCA Foods dressing*	*Italian Sausage w/onions, peppers & arugula salad*

SNACKS: *piece of LOCA Foods zucchini bread, LOCA Foods chocolate chip cookies*
BOWEL MOVEMENTS:
OVERALL MOOD:

Food Diary provided by LOCA Foods, LLC for Food as a Prescription - info@locafoodsinc.com

SAMPLE 2

FOOD DIARY

We recommend you use this #FoodDiary as a helpful tool on your journey. Visit our website at www.locafoodsinc.com to get a PDF emailed to you which you can print at home. While keeping track of your food throughout the day, be sure to also notate any liquids you consume and any environmental changes including new products you try.

Day 1 - Date: *Monday*

BREAKFAST *Time:*	**LUNCH** *Time:*	**DINNER** *Time:*
Homemade Chicken soup with rice ramen	*Grass-fed burger w/pepperoni, provolone, homemade honey mustard on gluten-free roll, a handful of chips and pickle chips*	*Chicken cutlet w/dairy-free mashed potatoes*

SNACKS: *LOCA Foods carrot cake*

BOWEL MOVEMENTS: **Include shape/texture as well as terms like constipation, normal, diarrhea*

OVERALL MOOD: **Include words like happy, stressed, content, sad, focused, balanced, etc*

Day 2 - Date: *Tuesday*

BREAKFAST *Time:*	**LUNCH** *Time:*	**DINNER** *Time:*
LOCA Foods Pancakes & 4 sausage links	*Chicken nuggets, a handful of honey mustard, handful of chips and a pickle*	*6 Tacos (Siete shells)*

SNACKS: *15 raw almonds, handful of gluten-free pretzels*

BOWEL MOVEMENTS:

OVERALL MOOD:

Day 3 - Date: *Wednesday*

BREAKFAST *Time:*	**LUNCH** *Time:*	**DINNER** *Time:*
ham, cheese & scallion omelette w/a pancake	*stuffed articoke*	*Grass-fed filet w/potatoes & onions w/LOCA Foods "no-corn" bread muffin*

SNACKS: *sesame seed cookies*

BOWEL MOVEMENTS:

OVERALL MOOD:

Day 4 - Date: *Thursday*

BREAKFAST *Time:*	**LUNCH** *Time:*	**DINNER** *Time:*
Frech toast w/maple sausages links	*Homemade chicken soup w/gluten-free egg noodles*	*Marinated grass-fed skirt steak w/non-dairy mashed potatoes & steamed carrots*

Food Diary provided by LOCA Foods, LLC for Food as a Prescription - info@locafoodsinc.com

Day 4 - Date: *Thursday*

BREAKFAST *Time:*	**LUNCH** *Time:*	**DINNER** *Time:*
Frech toast w/maple sausages links	*Homemade chicken soup w/gluten-free egg noodles*	*Marinated grass-fed skirt steak w/non-dairy mashed potatoes & steamed carrots*

SNACKS: *canteloupe pieces, LOCA Foods carrot cake slice*
BOWEL MOVEMENTS:
OVERALL MOOD:

Day 5 - Date:

BREAKFAST *Time:*	**LUNCH** *Time:*	**DINNER** *Time:*
NO BREAKFAST	*Gluten-free matzoball soup w/tinkyado shells*	*LOCA Foods lemon butter shrimp w/poached carrots*

SNACKS: *LOCA Foods chocolate cake slice*
BOWEL MOVEMENTS:
OVERALL MOOD:

Day 6 - Date:

BREAKFAST *Time:*	**LUNCH** *Time:*	**DINNER** *Time:*
Grass-fed steak & eggs	*Salami & ham on gluten-free bread w/safflower mayo, a handful of chips*	*Shared crab legs & LOCA Foods chicken wings w/lobster tail & rice*

SNACKS: *pasta salad, LOCA Foods chocolate chip cookies*
BOWEL MOVEMENTS:
OVERALL MOOD:

Day 7 - Date:

BREAKFAST *Time:*	**LUNCH** *Time:*	**DINNER** *Time:*
Frittata w/sausage, non-dairy cheese, peppers & onions	*NO LUNCH*	*Italian Sausage w/onions, peppers & arugula salad*

SNACKS: *banana, rice milk crunch bar*
BOWEL MOVEMENTS:
OVERALL MOOD:

Food Diary provided by LOCA Foods, LLC for Food as a Prescription - info@locafoodsinc.com

If you find this useful, print or download a PDF of your own at:

www.locafoodsinc.com

CHAPTER 8

CAREFULLY CRAFTED RECIPES

TO ASSIST YOU WITH this lifestyle, we are including six of our favorite go-to recipes we've developed over the past few years. We carefully crafted these recipes and, from the reviews, it is clear our friends and family love these dishes whether they are allergen-free or not. Ultimately, all we do is delicious. We hope you love them, or find ways to adjust the ingredients to work for you and your specific situation.

We'd like to start our recipe section by making you aware of an important staple in every kitchen: flour. Specifically, gluten-free flour—and even more specifically, a really, really good blend of gluten-free flours. We've spent a great deal of time and (way too much) money testing various types of individual and pre-mixed flours. After identifying which flours worked best, we could eventually successfully mix our own all-purpose flour. We haven't gone back to pre-made mixtures since! One of the major reasons we decided to explore mixing our own flour was because of the difference in expense. It's like anything else: if you do it yourself, it's often less expensive (and better!). You are welcome to use your own GF flour, but to get the best results, we highly recommend you utilize the GF flour mix we've included here.

Personal Tip: It's important to know that, as mentioned earlier, you cannot overmix gluten-free flour.

Make Your Own All-Purpose Flour Mixture (yield 4 C)

Depending on your specific sensitivities, you may need to adjust some of the flours to suit you. This will definitely change the consistency of the mix as well as anything you make with the new configurations. Just know, GF mixes can be very "moody".

Ingredients

2 C Almond Flour (sifted)
½ C Coconut Flour (sifted)
1 C Arrowroot Flour
½ C Tapioca Flour/Starch

Directions

1. Sift Almond Flour & Coconut flour into a large mixing bowl.
2. Add Arrowroot & Tapioca Flours.
3. Whisk together.
4. Make as much as you need and store in a cool/dry container/place.

Make sure you have a good sifter specifically made for flour. When storing your flour, use an air-tight container that is BPA-free (Bisphenol A).

Pancakes/Waffles

Ingredients

1 C GF flour mixture (use ours or any other that works for you)
1 Tbsp sugar (optional)
1 tsp salt
½ tsp baking powder
½ tsp baking soda
2 eggs (beaten)
½–⅓ C milk (choose your favorite alternative or traditional; we like walnut best for this recipe)
Splash of vanilla.

Directions

1. In a large glass measuring cup, add the dry ingredients and whisk together.
2. In a small glass measuring cup, beat the eggs and mix in the milk. *Ensure the liquid totals ¾ cup. (This total measurement of liquid varies depending on the milk you're using.) Then add vanilla and mix well.
3. Whisk liquid ingredients into dry until combined well.
4. Let batter stand while skillet/griddle is heating for about five minutes to allow it to thicken. Put your hand over the skillet/griddle; it should feel hot. If the mix is too loose, add additional tsp(s) of GF flour as appropriate. If mix is too solid, add additional milk or water as appropriate.

5. Pour batter into whatever size pancakes you desire. When batter starts to bubble a bit, flip. Cook until second side is done. Plate and enjoy.

If you have any batter left over, cover with plastic wrap and place in the refrigerator. This should last about three days, and we have personally found it to get better over time. When you remove it from the fridge, remove plastic and leave it to stand for 5–10 minutes. You may need to add a splash of water if the batter is a little thick.

Our Favorite Homemade Dressing (Mustard Vinaigrette)

Ingredients

1.5 Tbsp sugar (can reduce if need be)
3 Tbsp your favorite vinegar (we use coconut)
1 Tbsp Jewish "Deli" Mustard
2 cloves of garlic, minced
1/2 C extra virgin olive oil
1 medium shallot, finely chopped
Salt and pepper to taste.

Directions

1. Mix/whisk sugar and vinegar until sugar dissolves. Do not rush this step. You can let it sit and cut the garlic and shallot in the meanwhile.
2. Mix in the mustard.
3. Slowly whisk in the oil.
4. Mix in shallot, garlic, and salt and pepper to taste.
5. Refrigerate. (Be sure to remove from refrigerator about 15 minutes prior to using.)

Personal Tip: Get a salad dressing carafe and, after Step 1, put all ingredients into the carafe and shake vigorously to combine.

Dry Rub Chicken Wings

Ingredients

2 Tbsp tapioca flour
1 Tbsp maple sugar
½ Tbsp smoked salt
½ Tbsp onion powder
1 tsp garlic powder
1 tsp chili powder
½ tsp dry mustard
½ tsp cumin
¼ tsp rosemary (ground)
¼ tsp oregano (ground)
¼ tsp cinnamon

Additional dry ingredients:
2 Tbsp baking powder

Directions

1. Preheat oven to 250°F.
2. Line a baking tray with foil. Place baking rack on top and set aside.
3. Line a baking tray with foil. Place baking rack on top and set aside.
4. Line a baking tray with foil. Place baking rack on top and set aside.
5. Remove wings from the bag and place on baking rack evenly spaced.
6. Bake for 25 minutes, flip wings and bake for another 20 minutes.

7. Increase oven temp to 400°F. Bake for 20 minutes, flip wings and bake for another 15 minutes.
8. Remove from oven and set your oven to Broil at 500°F
9. Baste wings with your favorite GF BBQ sauce (we use our own "Slather Sauce"—one of the bonus recipes you can find at www.foodasaprescription.com).
10. Return basted wings to oven and broil for 3–5 minutes on a low rack.
11. Remove from oven, place in a bowl or on a plate and serve.

Lemon Butter Shrimp

Ingredients

16 jumbo (21/25) wild-caught shrimp cleaned and de-veined
2 eggs whisked
1 lemon halved and juiced separately
½ C LOCA Foods flour blend (from above)
1 tsp salt
½ tsp garlic powder
¼ tsp pepper
Oil for frying (coat pan 1/8") – something with a higher smoke point such as avocado or olive
¼ C non-dairy butter
¼ lb snow peas (or green beans)
¾ C broth of choice
¼ C water
¼ C DRY Ginger Ale
½ tsp salt
¼ tsp pepper
2 tsp arrowroot flour
1.5 tsp cold water

Directions

1. Whisk eggs and juice of ½ lemon together in a bowl then set aside.
2. Put flour, salt, garlic powder, and pepper in a large baggie. Shake to mix. Add shrimp and ensure all shrimp are coated in the mixture.
3. Heat 1/8" oil in a large skillet (cast iron preferred) on med-high heat.

4. Once oil is hot, dip each shrimp in egg mixture and transfer to hot pan. Flip after 2–3 minutes in batches if necessary.
5. Meanwhile, melt butter (alternative) in small pot. When melted, add snow peas (or green beans) & sauté 2–4 minutes tossing occasionally to ensure all sides are cooking. Then add broth, water, ginger ale, juice from other half of lemon, salt, and pepper and bring to a boil. Lower heat and add arrowroot mixture 1 tsp at a time until desired thickness. Remove from heat.
6. When shrimp are done frying, place on paper towel lined plate.
7. When sauce is to the thickness of your liking, plate shrimp on a bed of your favorite gluten-free pasta or rice and pour sauce over the top. Garnish with fresh parsley if desired.

Serves 2 people as written.

Chocolate Chip Cookies

Ingredients

1 C of butter softened OR 3/4 C (1.5 sticks) of Earth Balance (DF Alternative) (Soy Free)
1 C sugar
1 C maple sugar
2 eggs
2 tsp vanilla
3 C GF flour (from above)
2 tsp baking powder
1 tsp baking soda
1 tsp smoked salt
1/8 tsp cinnamon
1 C dark chocolate chips (Enjoy Life)
1 C semi-sweet mini chips (Enjoy Life)
1 C chopped walnuts

Directions

1. Cream the butter and sugar.
2. Crack eggs into a small bowl and whisk with vanilla, then add into the mixer.
3. In a separate bowl, combine flour, baking powder, baking soda, smoked salt, and cinnamon. Whisk and then slowly add to your batter.
4. Once batter has come together, stir in your chocolate chips and walnuts (if desired).
5. Chill dough for at least 5 hours.

To make a batch, preheat oven to 350° F. Once heated, spoon out portioned cookie dough on a tray covered with parchment paper. Make sure to leave room for them to spread. Bake for 18–20 minutes (the edges should start to get brown). We turn the tray around in the oven halfway through cooking.

When the cookies are done, allow to cool a few minutes before moving them from the cookie sheet to a wire rack.

We hope you enjoy preparing these recipes! Please take photos, tag us on any/all social media, and share your experiences with our foods. We look forward to seeing your results and hearing your stories!

You can use our Instagram (@locafoodsinc), our Facebook™ page (facebook.com/locafoodsinc and facebook.com/FoodRxBook), or our Twitter (@LOCAFoodsInc)!

Head over to the following link to get five more free recipes:

www.locafoodsinc.com

END NOTE

NOW THAT YOU HAVE read about our experiences and advice, we encourage you to formulate your own plan to apply food as a prescription. Use this book as a guideline for how you can devise a plan to live the rest of your allergen-free life. Ultimately, using your food as a prescription will help you to seek out what you need and to treat yourself with love and respect. Take your life back!

Don't be discouraged by others. Have confidence in your approach! You've got this, and if you ever need help, reach out to us, and we'll do everything in our power to help you help yourself. Best wishes on your journey!

If you liked this book, or if it helped you in any way, please tell others. We want as many people as possible to discover the benefits of using food as a prescription. Visit us at www.foodasaprescription.com for more information.

RESOURCES

Crowd Cow:
https://www.crowdcow.com/lu8zymt3xfqg

Green Tidings:
http://www.greentidings.com/discount/2f?redirect=%2F%3Fafmc%3D2f%26utm_campaign%3D2f%26utm_source%3Dleaddyno%26utm_medium%3Daffiliate

Anthony's Goods (flours):
http://www.anthonysgoods.com?afmc=di

Make your own Food Card here:
https://locafoodsinc.com/affiliates

Make your own Food Bag here:
https://locafoodsinc.com/affiliates

Butcher Box:
http://fbuy.me/qO2kw

Head on over to our website for even more of the amazing deals listed in this book to help you in using food as a prescription (www.locafoodsinc.com/affiliates).

ACKNOWLEDGEMENTS

Staci

I BELIEVE WE ARE all on a journey to find the best life we can while we are on this planet—however many times we may inhabit it. I have discovered how to strive for that in my life, thanks to a number of people I have encountered. I would like to acknowledge all those who have helped me on my journey. They include, but are not limited to:

My mother and family, for always listening, supporting, encouraging, helping, and loving me;

My husband and co-author of this book, Anthony, for his support in our continuing journey together, and for trusting me to always have our best interests at heart;

Any doctor whom I have seen in my lifetime, whether their philosophies were the same as mine or not;

All of my theatre friends for their encouragement in finding healing and to pursue my passion, whether or not I looked like the typical dancer/performer (along with remembrance of all the fun times we had!);

Every student who has pushed me to become the best teacher I can be at all times;

Every employer who has helped me to move forward in life's journey, and who have encouraged me to do whatever I needed in order to feel like and present my best self;

My #TapFam, for always being there and providing a safe space to exist and dance in;

Ben Gioia, for his guidance and motivation in helping Anthony and I to get this book out of our brains and onto paper;

Brad, for his friendship and always being willing to help with anything (including the new cover art!);

Hollie, for helping us get some documents in order;

Kelley and Amber, for so many things;

Rhonda for her kind editing suggestions;

And any reader of this book who is inspired to take charge of their health by using their food as a prescription.

I hope you use this book as a guide to help enjoy your journey and learn new things about yourself that lead to having the best Earthly experience possible.

Anthony

I care. I am a teacher at heart, and I want to leave the world knowing that I did everything in my power to help all humans—including myself—to become the best possible version of themselves. In line with this, I want to acknowledge the following:

Myself, for being willing to change;

My parents, for allowing me to have a lifestyle that opened me up to learning about life itself and, therefore, my own self;

My wife, Staci, for showing me this path;

Dr. Robert, for being one of those special people I have been lucky enough to know for almost my entire life;

Ben Gioia, for sharing his knowledge and energy with us;

Daria Walsh, for reminding me that she worked for a publisher;

Hayley Paige, for being that publisher, and for doing all the things a publisher does—plus all the things a good human does for other good humans;

Rhonda Foote, for jumping in and helping us get closer to the finish line;

Every teacher I ever had, for teaching me;

Every mentor I ever had, for mentoring me;

Tap dance, for the life lessons it has provided me with;

And, finally, anyone else who has believed in me, encouraged me, and supported me during my 48 years of life. Without you all, I may have never found my way to using food as a prescription.

Staci and Anthony are already working on their follow-up book to "Food as a Prescription" and have plans to publish, "All We Do is Delicious Vol.1: A Cookbook for Everyone — Including Those Who are Gluten-Free, Soy-Free, Corn-Free and Sometimes Dairy-Free".

www.ingramcontent.com/pod-product-compliance
Lightning Source LLC
LaVergne TN
LVHW010106110826
845155LV00028B/508
* 9 7 8 1 9 1 3 2 0 6 4 5 1 *